Can't Fry Me

Karen Lanso

Published by Karen Lanson

Copyright 2014 Karen Lanson

Introduction

Like most people I know all too well the euphoric high of losing weight followed by the inevitable, sooner or later crashing low of never maintaining the hard earned results.

This is something which can affect people regardless of their age, social status, gender or race. I have spent most of my life on or off a diet, obsessing about food and being in a love/hate relationship with my body. From childhood I struggled with my weight and spent a long time trying to make myself 'perfect.' Even as a fitness professional, common sense isn't and wasn't always so common, even to me. Explaining to someone why they shouldn't eat certain foods or should do more exercise to lose weight is like describing the water to a drowning man – in most cases people *know* what to do, they just don't know *how* to do it. Years of yo-yoing, wholeheartedly embracing the newest fitness fads (which are usually just revamped and repackaged programmes from an earlier time) only to achieve then all too quickly lose results is demotivating and tiring, mentally, physically and financially. Let's not forget that the diet industry is a multi million pound business empire which relies on people's failures in order to function! We have been given so many choices for health and fitness regimes all dangling that precious carrot of 'thin' that we are sometimes unable to make one. I remember the first time I was thin. A near starvation diet combined with grueling exercise seemed a small price to pay for the compliments and envious looks I received in abundance. Eventually I cracked. I was hungry! I was miserable and sick of calculating every morsel that passed my lips and being trapped in the same compulsive obsessive pattern day in and day out. I had been congratulating myself on my steely determination and self control when in fact my body demons had been controlling me all along. I decided to redress the balance and seize control of my life. After many false starts I finally *got it*, and kept it.

I know from my own personal experience the damage that those unwanted inches can have on your overall being. I developed a mild form of dysmorphia (sometimes referred to as *imagined ugliness* where the sufferer becomes obsessed with their appearance and minor or imagined flaws) and bulimia. I would behave like a fat girl in a skinny girl's body and vice versa. Think of a body con dress on a figure two stone overweight and you get the picture. Aside from the cosmetic gains which are usually the first motivator for people to turn to fitness, the health and mental benefits are huge. Most people will happily admit to being at their most beaming when they are at *their* ideal body shape, due to an increase in confidence, sense of achievement and improved health to list just a few of the reasons.

Can't Fry Me Love has come to fruition during my years of working within the fitness industry as an instructor, trainer and fitness model. It is a personal trainer in your pocket that will not blind you with science but simply addresses the most commonly (and repeatedly) encountered questions in the fitness and beauty world.

I have seen many people blossom from depressed, overweight, unhealthy beings into spriteful individuals with a zest for life. I am one of them. Many times I have witnessed people banishing health ailments by implementing positive changes and finding a new lease of life with a quality and gusto to it that they had never experienced before.

I hope you have as much fun reading this book as I did writing it.

Enjoy.

THE 'WEIGHT' IS OVER!

Dieting Makes You Fat

Absolute fact. The body can only burn up to 2 lbs of *fat* a week. Anything more than this is lean muscle tissue and water. Loss of muscle leads to a drop in metabolism which in turn slows down the rate at which the body burns calories. The faster you lose weight the less likely you are to maintain your results, and the harder it will become to lose weight in the future.

Our bodies are designed to cope in a 'desert' situation. Long inflicted spells of starvation will make your body cling onto and then convert into fat *any* food you give it as it prepares itself for future 'famine' in order to survive.

Tip: Breakfast really is the most important meal of the day (you are 'breaking' your 'fast' having not eaten for hours whilst sleeping.) The body slips into starvation mode after 4 hours of not eating.

Listen up serial yo-yoers! Crash dieting for that big event is not a good idea. You may well look fabulous in that little black dress, but I guarantee that you will go back to square one and then some when you return to your normal eating habits.

On a more serious level, extreme dieters who have spent years gaining then losing weight to only then repeat the cycle run the risk of laying down fat inside the internal organs which can pose much bigger problems than a muffin top. 'Visceral fat' is a dangerous fat which can heighten the risk of diabetes, heart disease and cancer. THE GOOD NEWS IS THAT IT IS NEVER TOO LATE TO CHANGE!

Consistency is key here. Make a decision right now to replace the word '*diet*' with '*healthy eating*.' Food is neither 'good' nor 'bad' and I believe that to refer to it in these terms simply reinforces negative behavior and creates a destructive relationship with it. Ditto banning any food group as this generates obsession which can then lead to rebellious bingeing. 'Forbidden Fruit Syndrome' – everything looks more desirable when you are not allowed to have it. Everything in moderation, food like everything in life should be enjoyed. However, what you do need to do is raise your awareness so that you can make informed choices. The *fact* here is that some foods will sate true hunger and some will generate further artificial hunger pangs.

I Can't Stop Comfort Eating

Like many addictions the way to conquer this is by *reprogramming* your mind and *relearning* habits. It is important to identify the *cause* in order to treat the *effect*.

Many behaviour patterns are established in childhood.

Like many people I associated treats with good times, like birthdays and Christmas. Freud believed that 'Oral Fixation' occurred as a result of a suckling baby taking either too much or too little pleasure in breastfeeding resulting in an obsession with 'comfort via the mouth' later on in life during times of stress, be it in the form of eating, smoking, nail biting or alcoholism.

We were told to eat everything on our plates, and if you didn't would maybe be made to feel guilty about the starving people in Africa or be told how loathsome it was to waste food after people had to ration during the wars. I'm not disputing that these are horrendous situations, but nor do I think that force feeding yourself is going to really salvage the problem. Your choice to eat when you're hungry then stop when you're full is unlikely to generate world peace or a redistribution of wealth! We can combat the problem of waste by being more aware of our portions. Learn how much is appropriate for you and then cook and buy the relevant amounts and store any remainders for another meal.

Many people no longer know how much is *truly* enough for them. We are used to feeling *hungry* which is good, as this means that we are sticking to our diet and are therefore losing weight, or *stuffed* which is bad because we've over done it, but we don't know (and need to learn) how it feels to be *satisfied.*

The most common reason for comfort eating is that we are using food to medicate another need or emotion such as stress, loneliness, sadness, boredom, or to reaffirm feelings of self loathing. You eat, enjoy a momentary high, feel like a failure, reinforce the negative image you have of yourself, think what the hell, you've ruined it now anyway, eat some more and so the circle continues. Your feelings are mirroring the science of what is happening in your body. The foods you eat when you comfort eat (I have never known anyone to binge on lettuce leaves and tuna) raise your serotonin and insulin levels (high) and then send them plummeting (low) which makes you want to repeat the cycle to raise yourself from the slump, both physically, emotionally and mentally.

Tip: Keep a food diary and *honestly* record everything that you eat and drink. Seeing something written down is a powerful way to raise your awareness and establish new patterns. Some people also find that keeping a photo journal of their meals is a good way to stay on track and helps with portion control. Ditto 'before' and 'after' body shots to track progress at regular intervals.

Humans are all predominantly the same in that we want to be happy, confident and have self respect which is acquired through *achievement* and fulfilling our *goals*.

So before you sit crying into that family size Dairy Milk, remember that you ARE NOT depriving yourself if you don't have it. You are choosing to NOT DEPRIVE yourself of looking and feeling the way that you want to.

Like any addiction take it a day at a time. Each day you put between you and 'it' gives you strength and distance. You will stop giving away your power and learn the difference between a little of what you fancy and a full blown binge. You don't have to do it all in one go. You just have to start.

Comfort Eating Is Making Me Fat

This isn't so 'duh' as it sounds. Obviously calorific foods laden with fat when consumed in large quantities are going to pile on the pounds. However, another contributing factor to take into account here is a substance called *'cortisol.'* This is a stress hormone produced in the adrenal gland which is created and released into the body when we are feeling stressed. Cortisol and adrenaline are released to help the body cope in a 'fight or flight' situation. In prehistoric times this would be for survival, i.e. hunting or fighting for your life. The adrenaline would make you alert and prepare you for oncoming battle and the cortisol would provide energy by increasing levels of fat and sugar into the bloodstream. Therefore you would be provided with and use the necessary fuel there and then. Unfortunately, these days stress is stress, and it makes no difference to your body if this is as a result of financial problems, domestic issues or day to day problems (external stress) or a rush of insulin from starch or sugar laden foods (internal stress) - the result on your body is the same. The body doesn't know that we have evolved from caveman times. If you were foraging for food or fleeing from a tiger as in the old days you would use the energy. These days, we don't burn the energy, we sit stewing in the car or at a desk or on the tube getting more and more stressed and creating more and more cortisol which in the absence of being used results in a band of fat around the abdomen.

This has been deemed the 'apple' shape for both men and women - a big midsection with smaller arms and legs. I have observed more and more apples in the last few years largely due to increased stress levels in day to day living but also an accumulation of bad habits due to hectic lifestyles.

Tip: A woman's waist measurement *across the navel* should be no more than 32 inches, and a man's should be no more than 37 inches.

Whilst adrenaline levels quickly return to normal, cortisol levels remain high sometimes for as long as a few days after a stressful event. Therefore, your body thinks it constantly needs to refuel to be able to cope with the fight or flight it expects as a result of receiving stress signals, and voila!

Stress = constant hunger!

We don't burn the energy and so it simply turns to fat. The fat goes to the waist because it is close to the liver and therefore can be easily burned as fuel if needed. On this token, any foods you comfort eat when stressed will also be attracted like a magnet to the middle of the abdomen.

It is so important for our body, mind and soul to de stress. Exercise is wonderful as it is connects you to the present moment through focus enabling you to detach from other issues. Alternatively, try a hot bath, read a book, watch a film or do anything that allows you to *disconnect* from the sometimes chaotic routines in which we live and *reconnect* with yourself.

Stress is literally a killer. It damages our internal matter and the results of this become visible on the outside. When you feel upset, angry or negative and someone asks you, 'What's the matter?' what they are seeing is the internal damage seeping through to your exterior (we are made of 'matter.') Everything truly comes from within.

Overweight people feel hungry all the time because their bodies are being deprived of and are therefore craving vital nutrients missing from unhealthy eating plans. It is possible to be obese and malnourished if you continually make poor food choices. If your car is running on empty and needs petrol, filling the tank with water will not salvage the problem however much you put in! Remember the 80 - 20 split, tow the line 80% of the time and give yourself 20% leeway.

I'm Too Depressed To Exercise

If you are prone to bouts of depression, all the more reason to exercise! As with all problems, there is a logical solution. Admittedly, it can be hard to always remain positive and 'be in the moment,' especially if the moment is on a crowded tube with a briefcase digging into your ribcage, unexpected expenses like the boiler breaking (all that money on something you can't even wear) traffic jams etc. etc. etc. The fact remains that stress is bad on many levels, therefore being happy is obviously good.

Simple but true.

Exercise produces *serotonin* - the same feel good hormone produced by chocolate and other starchy, sugary foods, only minus the negative impact on your figure and indeed your mind that inevitably follow a food binge. It is a scientific fact that exercising elevates your mood there and then, relieving feelings of stress and depression (they are often linked) and therefore eliminating the production of cortisol. Deep breathing is also instantly calming as it lowers the heart rate and removes the panic sensation which accompanies stressful situations. Pilates and yoga are good for learning and practicing relaxation and breathing techniques.

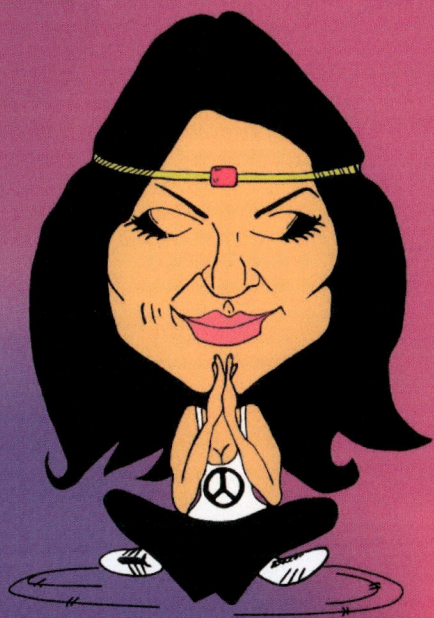

Kaz says...relax

I Haven't Got The Discipline And I Can't Be Bothered

In that case, you will just have to embrace life as an overweight, unhealthy and unhappy individual and like they say in New York, 'Get over it, and if you can't get over it, get over talking about it' (because you're driving the rest of us crazy!)

It's a slippery slope, I'll give you that - the less you do the less you want to do. Anything in life worth having requires some work and maybe a little sacrifice. If you want qualifications you study. If you want a relationship to work you invest in it. If you want an occasion to be successful you organise the factors to make it so. This is no different. There is *no* feeling like achieving your personal goals. You earn your stripe and quite rightly wear it as a badge of honour. Admittedly, only *you* can take that first step but then only *you* will reap the feel good benefits of your success! This sense of achievement will carry over into all areas of your life and you will feel more happy and confident because of it.

What we do have to do here is some serious damage control. It is your past negative, unsuccessful and non enjoyable experiences with health and fitness which have left you with the opinion that exercise and healthy eating are some kind of self imposed prison sentence.

On the contrary! The physical and almost *immediate* benefits (increased energy levels, improved health, better sleeping patterns, a more positive mindset to name but a few) brought about by small changes will leave you wondering why you didn't do it years ago.

Sweet Dreams!

7 - 8 hours of sleep is advised per night. This is when the body rejuvenates. Leptin, a chemical which curbs the appetite by suppressing the production of fat cells (also produced by strength training) is released into the body when you sleep. When sleeping time decreases, so too do your leptin levels resulting in cravings for starchy, sugary foods for that automatic 'hit' and to help you stay awake during the day. So just increasing your sleep time to at least 7 hours a night can help you lose weight!

For any insomniacs, milk when heated releases a hormone called melatonin which helps to induce sleep. It also contains L-tryptophan, an amino acid which has the same effect. A low fat hot chocolate with organic skimmed milk is a great way to get a 'sweet fix' minus the unwanted fat and calories.

Any snorers would benefit from losing weight as this is sometimes caused by excess pressure on the chest and by fatty deposits being laid down in the neck which restricts the breathing. In men, a neck measurement of more than 17 inches is dangerous. A condition called sleep apnea can also develop. This is when breathing stops completely and you have to awaken to regain a normal breathing pattern. This can not only be unpleasant at the time, but leads to daytime exhaustion due to interrupted sleep.

Pilates, yoga, or any other calming activity to calm and rest the mind will help if you have trouble switching off at the end of the day.

If I Stop Eating Carbohydrate At Night Will This Help Me To Lose Weight?

As long as you are burning more calories than you are consuming you will lose weight. However, when you sleep, it is the body's time to rejuvenate itself. Therefore it is more beneficial to eat a light dinner a few hours before you go to bed so that the body can replenish itself as you sleep rather than blood having to rush to the stomach to aid digestion. Carbohydrate when eaten earlier in the day is more likely to be burned as energy.

'Carbohydrate' is not the enemy. STARCH (bread, potatoes, rice and pasta) should be *monitored* for weight loss. As always, moderation is key, but it is easier to avoid constant hunger pangs when your insulin levels are not rocketing and plummeting due to a load of sugar being constantly dumped into your bloodstream.

Porridge oats and certain fruits and vegetables are carbohydrates but can be consumed without damaging your figure and also have amazing health benefits.

Tip: Learn how to 'spend' your daily calories wisely. As long as you come in at the given amount you will get results. Forward planning is required here. If you know that you are going out for a 3 course dinner then eat lightly at breakfast and lunch to balance it out.

I'll Always Be Fat

I interviewed an ex smoker. They gave up on many occasions with the aid of self help books, gum, willpower etc. Each time they would last an impressive few days before succumbing with an 'I'll try harder next time' attitude. After the first drag on the cigarette their sense of failure would come crashing down around them, and after the first hit which often made them feel dizzy and sick, they didn't enjoy the rest of the cigarette either but as they'd already poisoned their body and 'failed' in their mind, they would adopt a 'may as well be hung for a sheep as for a lamb' attitude and would finish the cigarette. And then another…and another.

Eventually, they realized that in order to succeed they would need to do something differently, but that *if they continued employing the same techniques then they would continue to get the same results.* So they modified their behaviour and avoided trigger points which they knew would tempt them when they were feeling vulnerable. They didn't go out to pubs or clubs (which they assosciated with smoking) until they felt that they had a sufficient amount of time between themself and their addiction. They had tea in the morning instead of the cup of coffee that they used to enjoy with the first of their many cigarettes of the day. It's harder to throw away a week's work then an hour's work! When they did venture out again, they initially took a vice in the form of tabs which they no longer use either. They didn't want to be exiled socially and so suggested to friends that instead of going drinking they went to the cinema or to a class or just tried something new generally which opened up new opportunities and experiences for all of them.

Tip: The definition of insanity is repeating the same behaviour and expecting different results.

The feeling of self respect and achievement you earn when you conquer your demons is tremendous and carries over into all areas of your life. Success breeds success. This same mindset can be applied to food and all other bad habits or addictions. In rehabilitation clinics sufferers of food disorders are treated alongside people suffering from drug and alcohol abuse. Food is a legal drug but no less fatal if abused.

You can do anything you set your mind to. There may be moments when it's challenging, but quite frankly, if you want to make an omelette you have to break a few eggs! Cravings like anything in life are momentary and will pass.

The pros far outweigh the cons. You can do it!

Tip: 5 factors which affect weight loss are:Nutrition, Exercise, Hydration, Sleep and Hormones.

'I Can Resist Everything Except Temptation.'

Oscar Wilde, Playwright, Novelist and Poet

How many times have you fancied a chocolate bar and decided to abstain for the sake of being 'good?' So you have some crackers instead to be healthy. This doesn't quite scratch that itch, so you have some nuts. You're still not satisfied, and decide to be a little bit naughty. So you have some crisps. Until finally, you succumb and have a chocolate bar (on top of the crackers, nuts and crisps that you didn't even want.) As you've already been 'naughty' you decide to finish anything and everything chocolate/sugar/starch related in the house. After all, out of sight is out of mind and then you can start your diet again tomorrow…sound familiar? Don't worry - you're not alone. With true food cravings, the more you resist, the more they persist. Have what you want in the first place and save time and calories! A chocolate bar (or whatever floats your boat) when eaten and *enjoyed in moderation* is absolutely fine. The problems arise when you are using food in a mindless manner to fill another void. If you are going to eat, *enjoy it*, and then move on with your life without a backward glance. If not, just say no!

The Gym Is Making Me Fat

This reminds me of the joke when a woman asks her partner 'Does this dress make my bum look big?' to which he replies 'No, but all that chocolate and ice cream you keep eating does!'

Ladies, stop giving away your power! Try not to put people, including yourself, in an awkward lose lose situation by asking others to reaffirm what you can see for yourself. If you've had to shoehorn yourself into your jeans, chances are that you are *not* at your svelte best. It is also advisable not to weigh yourself in these circumstances as the chances that you have lost 10 lbs are slim, no pun intended. Stay focused and brace yourself for the compliments that will come flying your way when you *do* reach your goal!

Tip: Visualisation can be a very powerful tool. Use a picture of a body you admire (even a previous picture of yourself) that you want to achieve. Look at it often. Start *thinking* as the slim you right now. This will make you *behave* like the slim you right now.

A familiar pattern is that people reward their physical efforts with food post workout, for example by treating themselves to a take away and some wine after a session on the treadmill.

To lose weight you have to create a deficit whereby more calories are being burned than consumed. You may well be burning 400 - 600 calories when you train (depending on the activity, intensity etc.) However, if you then consume the same amount or more calories than you are burning, you will maintain your current weight or even gain more. Here's some food for thought…80% of appearance is down to *nutrition.* All the training in the world will not alter your appearance if your food habits are not adjusted accordingly.

Tip: Include weight training in your programme. When you do resistance training the body produces a protein called leptin which acts as an appetite suppressant. Strength training also increases bone density which reduces the risk of osteoporosis. Muscle is a furnace that burns fat, so the more muscle you have the more fat you will burn, even when you are sleeping.

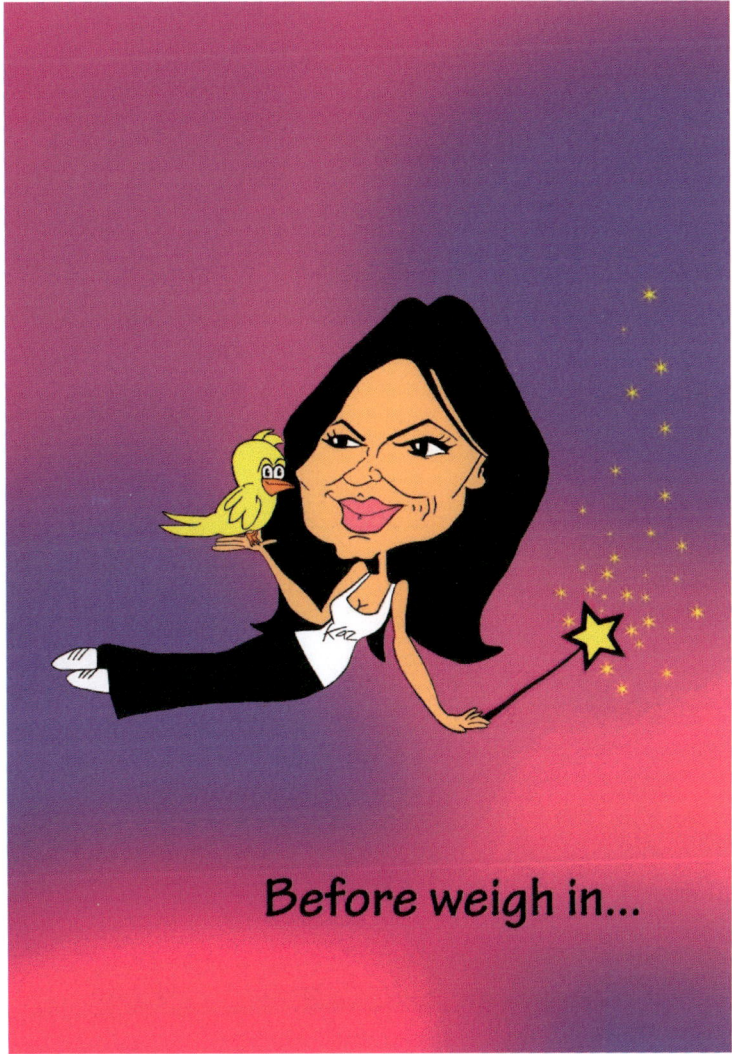

Before weigh in...

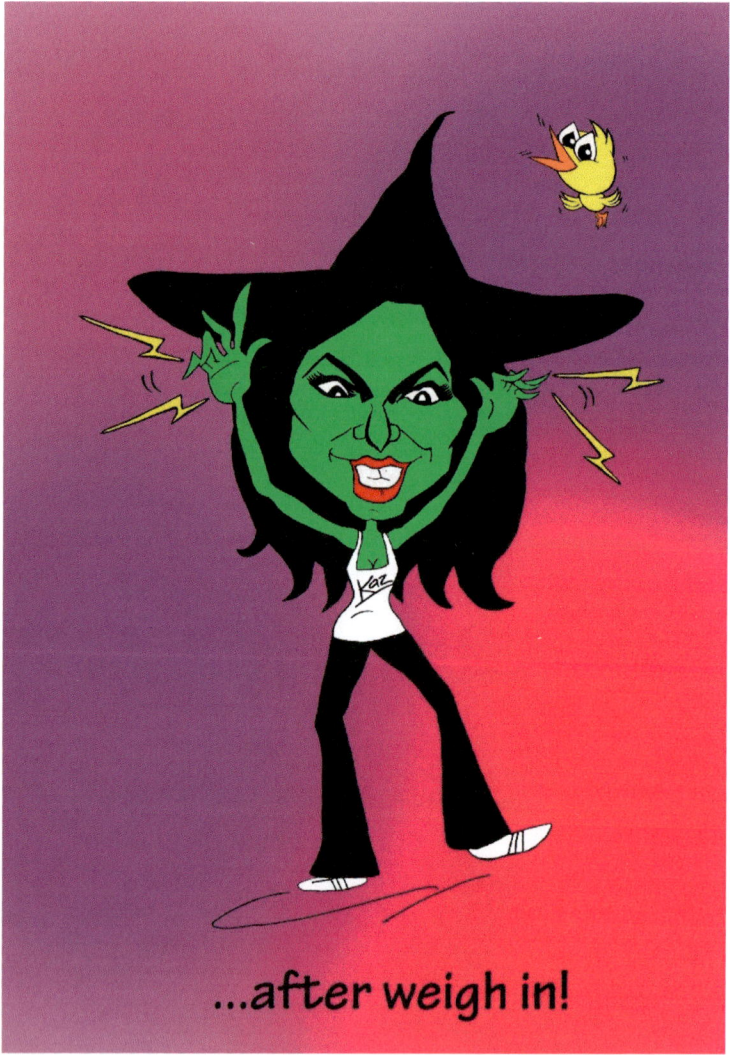

...after weigh in!

I Hate the Gym

'If God had wanted me to bend over he would have put diamonds on the floor.'

Joan Rivers, American Comedienne.

I know that some days it's harder to motivate than others, and this coupled with the fact that you hated your training would have you diving back under the duvet in no time.

Aerobic (working the heart and lungs) activity occurs when the pulse is raised and maintained.

60 - 70% of the maximum heart rate for fat burning

70 - 80% of the maximum heart rate for cardio training

Tip: 220 - Age = Maximum Heart Rate.

Aerobic activity should be performed 3 - 5 times a week, for a duration of 30 - 45 minutes per session.

Tip: A 'feast or famine' approach to exercise (intense spells of grueling training followed by bursts of inactivity) will have the same effect on the body as yo yo dieting. The body will switch to starvation mode in order to survive making it hard to burn fat and sculpt muscles. Make your fitness routine realistic for your lifestyle.

All of the following activities when performed at a moderate to vigorous intensity are aerobic:

Running, power walking, rowing, cycling, dancing (all

styles) football, volleyball, basketball, boxing, cheerleading, athletics, squash, and martial arts to name but a few.

Please note that a casual stroll around a golf course and chatty tennis matches do not count! You have to earn your shower! Anything is *not* better than nothing when working out - you do have to WORK!

Classes are fantastic. Connecting with others and building a social support network can be hugely beneficial for your health and fitness goals. You are learning and having fun in a class environment which stops you from getting bored and it helps to keep you motivated, plus you can relate to people who know what you are going through and what you are planning to achieve. Some people prefer to train alone doing their own routine or with a DVD or personal trainer. That's cool too. There is no right or wrong and one size never fits all. Ultimately, the most successful programmes are the ones that people stick to, so if you are enjoying your training you are halfway home. Find your 'thing' and do it.

Tip: The body and mind are intricately linked. Movement develops the body *and* the brain. Slow, cross lateral (working the left and the right side of the body in unison) integrated movements featured in yoga, tai chi and Pilates engage *all* areas of the brain. As a result, studies have shown dramatic results in children with ADD (Attention Deficit Disorder) ADHD (Attention Deficit Hyperactivity Disorder) and other learning disabilities who exercise. Exercise generates discipline, self control and self respect. A healthy body equals a healthy mind. More and more research is proving that degenerative diseases like Alzheimer's can be prevented simply by developing the frontal lobe of the brain which controls fine motor coordination, so a hobby like playing a musical instrument would be beneficial as a more sophisticated hand eye coordination is required. Learning is good for us! A substance called dopamine is released in the brain which gives us a 'spark' or zest for life which awakens our natural curiosity and a desire to learn more. Our confidence is increased and we become happier.

I Train Every Day, Watch What I Eat And Sill Haven't Lost *Weight!* Why?

Overtraining could be a factor. If you do the same routine repeatedly, regardless of the intensity, your body will simply adjust or *plateau* and progress will stabilise. What's needed here is to create *'muscle confusion'* - a shock to the body to restart progress. In this case, less is definitely more, and I would advise initially less weekly sessions (minimum of three) with higher intensity. *Quality, not quantity.*

Tip: To lose weight, *women* should consume 1500 calories a day (normally 2000)

Men should consume 2000 calories a day (normally 2500)

ANYTHING LESS WILL PUT THE BODY INTO STARVATION MODE.

Interval sessions are perfect for this as you alternate between your anaerobic and resting heart rate zones. Work flat out for a minute recover, repeat. This enables you to put 100% effort into the bursts as they are far more achievable when broken down into smaller sections and you are allowed time to catch your breath in between. In these instances a 20 minute workout is effective – in addition always remember to warm up, cool down and stretch post work out.

Overtraining is a waste of time, wear and tear on your body and motivation. You will be keeping up your *fitness* levels but if weight and inch loss are your super objectives then adjustments need to be made in order to achieve this. I would also advise that you resist the urge to weigh yourself at every available opportunity.

Tip: 5 lbs of muscle is approximately the size of 1 clenched fist. 5 lbs of fat is approximately the size of 4 clenched fists.

If you must, only ever use the same set of scales as results can vary causing confusion and frustration. Focus more on inch loss as fat takes up more room but muscle is heavier. A ton of feathers weighs the same as a ton of lead – they both weigh a ton! A more accurate way to monitor progress is to do a weekly trouser test. This is a much better way to gage how you're doing - the tape measure doesn't lie! However, scales often register no initial difference in your weight due to building muscle even when you have lost inches and they also don't take into account what is skeletal, muscle, fat or water weight.

Remember, if you are growing your hair, you don't scrutinise it daily observing every nth of an inch of growth. You simply go about your business until it is long enough to style as you wish, and it's the same principal here.

Tip: Set mini goals and reward yourself each time you

achieve one. Book a beauty treatment, go shopping, see a show…anything that makes you feel good! You are sending a powerful message to your subconscious that you value yourself and are worthy of wonderful things as you are *now,* not just when you can rock your skinny jeans.

I've Been Exercising And Eating Healthily For Weeks And Still Haven't Lost Weight Or Inches! Why?

In the same way that you don't just *suddenly* (unless you have medical issues) put on weight, if you want to *maintain* your results you cannot just suddenly lose it either. A single packet of biscuits when binge eaten won't render your entire wardrobe unwearable. 10 will. 1 glass of wine won't force you out of every pair of tailored trousers you own and into sweatpants. 5 bottles might.

If you think honestly, it's an accumulation of *bad habits* built up over a *period of time* that have caused the problem in the first place. If you have spent a lifetime sending your body mixed messages (1 minute there's a food shortage, the next you are eating anything and everything) it will take *time* for your body to readjust to your new life. Patience is compulsory here as this is the hardest part. Instant gratification doesn't work which we know from the 'lose 20 lbs in 2 weeks' gimmicks. In my experience in general, anything that sounds too good to be true usually is. You may not see it, but it *is* working. Many a time, clients have threatened to throw in the towel having not seen physical changes after a few weeks, even though their energy levels had rocketed, they were sleeping better and were generally more upbeat and healthier. They stuck with it, and in such cases, people would lose a few pounds all in one go. Once through the initial barrier, weight loss would stabilise at a steady 1 - 2 lbs a week. Hang tough. Don't throw the towel in - use it to wipe your sweat and then get back to your workout!

The 'Chunky Aerobic' Syndrome

People who undertake large amounts of aerobic exercise *only* often note that in spite of long, sweaty sessions they cannot seem to shift unwanted body fat or build lean muscle mass and look 'chubby.' The main cause for this is because cardiovascular work produces very little elevation of metabolism once the exercise has stopped. In other words, the minute the session ends, the metabolism muscle cells stop burning extra energy. Strength training on the other hand due to increasing the size of muscle cells (which are fat burning machines) keeps the metabolism burning energy for 3 - 4 hours once the session has ended! This in turn will burn fat and unwanted calories long after you have finished training! Yippee!

I Don't Want To Do Weights, I'll Bulk Up

I have found this to be a common cause for concern amongst women, and one that is completely unfounded. Women do not have the same testosterone levels as men, so an 'Arnie Body' would be hard to achieve based on the 'high repetition, low weight' formula that is employed in most classes and training environments anyway. The women you see in some commercial bodybuilding magazines and competitions have adjusted their training and eating regimes deliberately to achieve muscle mass and in extreme (not all) cases assistance has also been obtained from substances to achieve the physiques that they have.

Tip: Always stretch your muscles after training. Muscles shorten when they are worked so stretching will lengthen them and realign the fibres. This will not only help to avoid injury but will promote a sleek, elongated silhouette.

Cellulite! Help!

Expensive creams and treatments are fine, but I have found that the best remedy for cellulite is *dry body brushing*. This is one of the beauty world's best kept secrets! Invest in a body brush and in circular motions starting at the feet, work upwards (avoid your décolletage as the skin is very delicate in this area) and go towards the heart so as not to disrupt the blood flow and cause thread veins. Do this daily to kick-start the lymphatic drainage system (the body's natural waste removal system.) Try and cut down on alcohol, smoking, processed food, sugar and caffeine as these all cause toxins which are deposited in the body resulting in cellulite. Increase your intake of water to flush toxins through the body. You will also notice an improvement in skin tone and texture. Deep tissue massage helps and also aids muscle recovery post workouts.

Dress For 'The *Weigh'* You Are

There are three general body types (somatotypes) which are:

Mesomorphs

This body type is referred to as 'athletic.' Think Britney Spears and Madonna for the girls, Bruce Willis and

Arnold Schwarzenegger for the boys.

Ectomorphs

Willowy with very little body fat. Think catwalk models. Kate Moss for the girls and Brad Pitt for the boys.

Endomorphs

Short, rounded and pick up weight easily. It's not all bad news though - the most famous endomorph of all time is still hailed as a sex siren today. Marilyn Monroe.

People are often a mix of somatotypes, and may have characteristics from more than one, for example a *meso - endomorph* may be predominantly muscular but with a tendency to gain fat easily. Genetics do come into play here, but once again forewarned is forearmed! Generally, fat burning is fat burning but strength and toning work can be modified to suit the individual shape. A whole body approach is always advisable for balance and overall health.

Your body shape is deciphered by hormones. Whilst it is difficult to spot reduce specific areas you can influence your workout by tricking these hormones into burning body fat from required problem zones with these two simple tips.

1) Do some strength training prior to your cardio session to 'rev up' your metabolism.

2) Drink a cup of black coffee pre workout. Caffeine stimulates the nervous system which in turn sends signals to the fat cells to break down fat. Drink PLENTY of water before, during and after training as caffeine is a

diuretic.

Of course these somatotypes are referring to people in their *natural* body state, not when they are severely under or overweight. Our body *will* alter slightly during the course of our life, particularly at certain times of the year like Christmas or maybe during holiday periods. Even though we know the sizing in clothes is not 100 per cent reliable, I would advise that if you do fluctuate on these occasions to *not* buy clothes bigger than your normal size. This sends yourself the message that you are accepting the situation and have resigned yourself to it. Instead, focus on your skin, hair, manicures and pedicures to keep yourself looking and feeling good. The fact is, as you lose inches and your body shape changes, your fashion choices also alter to suit your new physique. For example, if you have been hiding under loose tops and dresses, when you have a sleeker silhouette it is only natural that you will want to show it off in more fitted clothes. There is no right or wrong here as fashion is a fabulous way to express yourself, but here are some handy ageless tips:

Apply fake tan. This makes you look instantly slimmer and highlights muscle definition. Subtle – not 'tango.' Healthier for your skin than long sunbathing sessions and DEFINITELY safer than sunbeds.

Bootcut, flared and wide legged trousers flatter most body shapes and balance the lower and upper body.

Outfits can be cinched in at the waist with a belt (or add a splash of colour with a scarf) for an hourglass shape.

Black opaque tights or hold ups make legs look amazing when worn with shorts or mini skirts. Legs appear to go on forever, especially if you add heels or wedges.

Highlight the areas you do like. Try to avoid drowning yourself in yards of fabric as this actually makes you look bigger. If you are wearing a floaty top like a kaftan, wear something fitted on the lower body and vice versa.

If you are wearing a revealing top, cover up your lower body to avoid showing too much flesh. Vice versa.

Make sure that you are wearing the right size bra, especially if your body shape has recently changed. This is one exception to the 'don't buy until you are the size you want to be' rule! Get measured and fitted correctly.

Dress in clothes that you feel comfortable in and suit your shape, regardless of the fashion at the time. You can update your look instantly with accessories and new shades of makeup.

It's not what you wear; it's how you wear it!

How Much Is Enough?

Portions. Okay, so no one has the time nor the inclination to measure every single morsel that goes into their mouth. Nor do we want to obtain a math degree simply to calculate our daily meal's allowance!

A helpful tip is to imagine your plate as a clock face. 1 -

4, protein (fish, quorn/soya/tofu) 4 - 6 starch/carbohydrate (brown rice, potatoes, pasta) 6 - 11, vegetables or salad, 11 - 12 essential fat.

Remember that your stomach is the size of your fist and that should guide you in the right direction. You could also try using a smaller plate. Chew your food thoroughly as enzymes released through saliva when chewing aid digestion which actually begins in the mouth, not the stomach. It also stops you from swallowing air which causes bloating. Men need more food than women, so ladies if you are the allocated cook your portion should be slightly smaller. If you are hungry eat, but try to avoid 'empty' junk calories with no nutritional value. Fill up on fruit and vegetables which are fibrous and contain water so that you can sate your hunger and thirst at the same time.

I'm Too Old To Start Exercising!

Tip: After 25 you get the face and body you deserve!

Many illnesses such as coronary heart disease, strokes, high cholesterol, diabetes, osteoporosis, arthritis and cancers to name but a few are not just exclusive to 'elderly people.'

Okay, so it *is* true that after 25 years old the body loses approximately half a pound of muscle tissue yearly, and we replace old bone cells less rapidly after approximately 35 years old, but once again, the great news is that EXERCISE and HEALTHY EATING can dramatically reverse the effects of 'ageing' and improve the quality of your life regardless of your biological age. Look at it this way; you just need to start/maintain doing what you should be doing anyway.

Exercise increases the production of synovial fluid in the joints which makes them more mobile and is therefore excellent for people with arthritis who have stiff joints. Exercises should be performed in a controlled manner to avoid the risk of injury, but that's a hard and fast rule generally when exercising.

Though genetics play a part, I believe that it is nurture and not nature that makes the ultimate difference. Think of it as forewarned being forearmed. For example, if you know that heart disease runs in your family, make a conscious decision to exercise regularly (the heart is a muscle - use it or lose it) and eat a good varied diet that's not too high in calories or saturated fat. This will also keep your cholesterol level healthy. Make this as compulsory to your everyday routine as brushing your teeth.

Start reading food packets and become aware of GDA (Guideline Daily Amount) and ingredients. Generally, if you can't pronounce it, don't buy it as the product is likely to be high in additives and preservatives and empty in nutritional value.

Tip: Low *fat* foods have 3g or less per 100g. Low *sugar* foods have 5g or less per 100g. Beware of 'low fat foods' which are higher in sugar and riddled with additives, and 'junk foods' masquerading as a healthy option.

Exercise should always be modified to suit the individual, and it should be fun. It doesn't have to mean pounding away on the treadmill for hours on end. Any instructor worth their salt will give you alternatives to take into account injuries or health conditions.

Many heart patients feel nervous returning to exercise

after an episode, but the sooner a graduated exercise programme is reintroduced the better. As well as the physical benefits, they will feel so much happier being back in control due to an increase in self confidence and a reduction in stress levels.

Osteoporosis is a weakening of the bones. It can affect anyone, but post menopausal women are highly at risk due to hormonal changes. Severely underweight women are also susceptible due to the withdrawal of hormones should their menstrual cycle stop. Once again, exercise to the rescue, as weight bearing exercise improves bone density helping to combat this. Weight bearing work will also build muscle tissue which keeps the body strong and lean. If you are vulnerable to osteoporosis, also work on your balance and overall stability. Minimise your risk of falling over to avoid fracturing your bones. Again, development of the frontal lobe in the brain raises alertness so that if you were to trip you could be more likely to steady yourself and less likely to fall.

Tip: Vitamin D is an advisable supplement for sufferers, as is calcium. Go easy on animal products such as red meat and cheese (reducing this will also lower cholesterol levels and will prevent artery blockage in the heart.) Arthritic patients also benefit from cutting down on animal products as they cause acidity in the joints. The *main* types of arthritis are osteo, rheumatoid (both 'wear and tear') and psoriatic. Animal protein, along with fizzy drinks and high levels of salt upset the acid balance in the body and calcium stores can then be depleted as the body takes calcium from the bones to neutralise the acid, weakening the bones. Watch your alcohol intake and generally aim to make your body alkaline.

Eat Young And Beautiful!

Too much refined sugar and carbohydrate not only raises blood cholesterol and piles on weight, it also destroys collagen in the skin resulting in wrinkles!

Tip: Vitamins A, C, D and E, are antioxidants which repair skin so eat a diet rich with these nutrients. Omega 3 oils are excellent for the skin and heart. Hair loss could be due to hormonal changes or a deficiency in vitamin B12 and iron. Vitamins B2, C and E are also advisable for a full, shiny head of hair.

Use a sun block, and avoid the sun approximately between 11 - 3 when the rays are at their strongest. Use a high SPF (sun protection factor) which protects against UVA (ageing) UVB (burning) and UVC (cancer.) Sun creams have life spans so remember to replenish them regularly and use them within their shelf life once opened. The sun does have health benefits too and because the ultra - violet rays trigger vitamin D synthesis in the skin it is also a known mood elevator, proven by people who suffer from S.A.D (Seasonal Affective Disorder) in the winter due to lack of sun and daylight.

Growing up is compulsory. Growing old is optional!

Calcium

Calcium has many nutritional benefits. It has been proven to reduce high blood pressure and the risk of colon cancer. It's high in protein and amino acid which builds and repairs lean muscle tissue. It is vital for bone health, and (drum roll please) it aids weight loss through the breakdown of fat! It gets better still. An expanding waistline is both frustrating and very ageing. This can occur in latter life due to hormonal changes within the body. Another well noted client concern is that people wish to lose weight without becoming 'haggard' in their facial appearance. When you have an eating plan rich in calcium but low in fat, BELLY FAT IS BURNED FIRST!

Tip: The recommendation is 1000 mg of calcium daily for pre menopausal women. This daily dosage should increase to 1500 mg for post menopausal and pregnant or nursing women. The body can only absorb 500 mg at any one time.

Vitamin D assists the body in absorbing calcium, whilst iron, fibre and caffeine stop the body fully absorbing calcium.

This Sounds Great But I Am Lactose Intolerant (Allergic To Dairy Products!)

Whilst dairy products, particularly low fat yoghurt (probiotic yoghurt also helps to maintain a healthy digestive and immune system and increases calcium absorption in the body, plus it contains 'good' bacteria) and low fat cheese remain good sources of calcium, there are other alternatives.

'The Pagoda' (Chinese Food Guide) lists the following food options:

Almonds, bok choy, broccoli, kale, salmon and sardines (though the bones must be consumed as that is where the calcium is found) and sesame seeds.

Some soy is an alternative – read the label - and is also high in protein. Try edamame beans which provide vitamins A and B, and some dairy intolerant people are able to consume goat's milk as a substitute for cow's milk.

Tip: 700g/ 1 lb 9 oz broccoli = 225ml/8 fl oz of skimmed milk. You have to consume a lot more vegetables to get the same calcium benefit provided by dairy products but it can be done and is far more ethical. As a vegan would ask, 'If you wouldn't give cow's milk to a new born baby than why would you give it to yourself?' Interesting point.

Mineral water also contains calcium.

Is It Me Or Is It Hot In Here?

Hot flashes, night sweats, vaginal dryness, mood swings, depression, weight gain, fatigue…hardly the stuff dreams are made of but the menopause is an inevitable part of every woman's life. However, more and more research is showing that all of the mentioned symptoms are actually more as a result of ageing than a direct result of the menopause itself, which is excellent news because it means that it can, to a certain degree, be controlled by the individual.

The WHI (Women's Health Initiative) in the States conducted a $625 million dollar study radical at the time (radical because a group of volunteers literally let the toss of a coin decide whether or not they would take oestrogen or be in a placebo group to determine whether or not it was truly beneficial during menopause at a time when HRT was the *only* option.) *Lifestyle (*exercise, good nutrition and a positive attitude) proved to be the most beneficial factor in reducing symptoms of the menopause. However, different strokes for different folks and to each their own. The average menopause starts at 51 and lasts for 4 years but affects everyone differently. HRT (Hormone Replacement Therapy) prescribed by the doctor *is* beneficial for some women. There are also herbal, plant based supplements which mimic the oestrogen produced by the body. It is down to the personal choice and preference of each individual, there is no right or wrong. Both forms carry a small risk as most things in life do, but people are more able to make an *informed* decision when they have all the *facts*. A diet high in soy is also thought to help as soy is a distant chemical relative of oestrogen. Cutting back on caffeine, alcohol and spicy foods can also help to reduce flashes and acupuncture is said to be beneficial. This time too will come to pass, and the end of your menopause is the start of your new life!

Tip: Do something every day that your future self will thank you for.

Don't Break Your Heart!

Saturated (animal) and **trans** (found in foods containing hydrogenated vegetable oil) **fats clog the arteries in the heart and elevate bad cholesterol levels.**

Mono and polyunsaturated fats lower bad cholesterol levels.

HDL Cholesterol = High Density Lipoprotein cholesterol which is GOOD.

This protects against heart disease.

Levels should be greater than 65 in women and 55 in men.

LDL Cholesterol = Low Density Lipoprotein cholesterol which is BAD.

This blocks the arteries.

Levels should be less than 130 mg/dl and less than 100 for cardiac rehab patients.

I feel it compulsory to mention at this point that 50 per cent of people with heart disease have normal cholesterol levels.

For excellent heart health, *reduce* your intake of trans and saturated fat, avoid excess alcohol, caffeine and sodium (salt) which all raise blood pressure, and also reduce refined carbohydrate and sugar. Smoking also clogs the arteries.

Increase fibre found in cereal, fruit and vegetables which will aid the body in processing and eliminating cholesterol. Fresh fruit and vegetable also provide potassium, another natural 'heart medicine.' Vitamin E is an anti-oxidant and great for circulation. Nuts and seeds are excellent sources of Omega which is vital for .your heart. Alternate red meat with fatty fish (also high in Omega) and poultry.

A healthy eating plan and regular exercise will also address any blood pressure issues. Blood pressure is recorded with a systolic reading (pressure when the heart contracts) and a diastolic reading (pressure when the heart relaxes.) This should be no higher than 140/90 and approximately on or at 120/80 in a healthy individual. The systolic reading varies depending on many contributing factors, such as stress, energy levels, whether you have consumed caffeine, alcohol etc. The diastolic reading is generally more consistent, and therefore the one that is monitored.

Tip: 95% of heart attacks which occur whilst exercising happen in the first 5 minutes so *always* warm up thoroughly for 5 - 10 minutes.

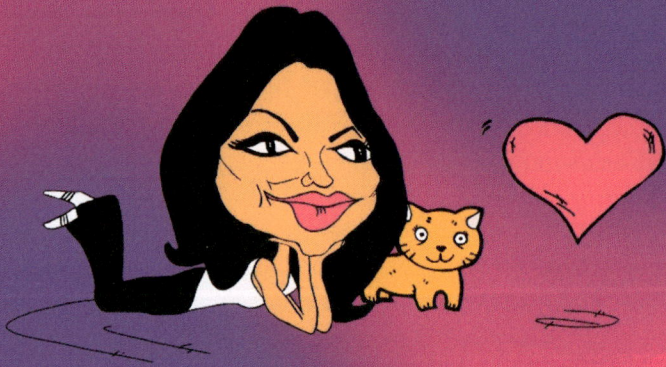

Love your heart...

The 'C' Word

'Cancer is a disease of the mind, body and spirit. A proactive and positive spirit will help the cancer warrior be a survivor. Anger, unforgiving and bitterness put the body into a stressful and acidic environment. Learn to have a loving and forgiving spirit. Learn to relax and enjoy life.' *John Hopkins Hospital*

Food and exercise are once again Mother Nature's prescription here.

Reduce/eliminate animal protein, processed food, alcohol and additives.

Increase beta carotene (the body converts this into vitamin A which is an antioxidant. The brighter the fruit or vegetable, the higher the beta carotene content.) Also increase your intake of vitamin C to strengthen the immune system and include oily fish, avocado and nuts for their Omega 3 fatty acid benefit.

Listed below are just some of the super foods which have cancer fighting properties:

Apricots, beetroot, blueberries, carrots, cherries, cranberries, grapes, lemons, limes, oranges, peppers, pomegranates, prunes, pumpkin, radishes, red cabbage, spinach, squash, swede, sweet potatoes, tomatoes, and watercress.

Everyone should aim for 5 (ideally 9) portions of fruit and vegetables daily.

Another highly dangerous chemical to be aware of is called **dioxin**. This causes cancer, particularly breast. If you are using a microwave and having a ready meal remove it from the carton and use a glass or microwaveable dish instead. I am personally not a fan of microwaves. They were banned at one point in Russia in 1976 due to their negative health connotations. If you wouldn't give a baby microwaved formula, why would you give yourself microwaved food? It's an ongoing debate, some for, some against. To each their own. Never drink from bottled water that has been left in the sun.

High heat + plastic = **dioxin** release into your food.

Also be aware that **dioxin** is released when plastic is frozen, so avoid putting plastic bottles in the freezer.

A low G.I. (Glycaemic Index) eating plan is a good idea for everyone. Due to the foods stabilising blood sugar levels the adrenal system is not overworked due to sudden insulin rushes (bought about by refined sugars and carbohydrates.) You also feel fuller for longer because of this so energy slumps and cravings are zapped. This is excellent for your long term health in general.

Strokes

Medical researchers have advised that the quicker a stroke is identified (usually within 3 hours) the higher the chances are of a neurologist being able to reverse the effects. The majority of strokes are caused by a blood clot in the brain. The sooner drugs (tPA) can be administered to break the clot allowing oxygen to flow freely to the brain, the sooner the damage can be stopped and reversed.

To identify whether or not someone has had a stroke, ask them to perform the following activities. Inability to do these could indicate a stroke. Remember the first 3 letters:

S - Ask the person to *smile.*

T - Ask the person to *talk* and speak a simple sentence, for example 'My name is ...'

R - Ask the person to *raise* both arms.

Also ask the person to *stick out their tongue.* If it is crooked or goes to the side, this could be another indication of a stroke.

Whilst I agree that little changes make big differences and that we should all aim to be more active in general, please note that walking up and down the stairs a couple of times a day does not a workout make. The heart rate has to be raised and then maintained for 30 - 45 minutes to constitute an aerobic session. Start off slowly and gradually increase your time and intensity. If you have or have had any serious medical conditions, are pregnant or have just given birth, consult a doctor before you begin training – and in most cases you will find that exercise is just what the doctor will order! Stop if you need to whilst training and rejoin the programme when you are ready but keep your feet moving (march on the spot, tap your toes etc.) so that you don't get blood rushing from your head to your feet (pooling) causing dizziness. Always keep yourself hydrated before, during and after training.

Tip: You can tell if you are drinking enough water by the colour of your urine - it should be clear and straw coloured. Any trace of yellow shows dehydration so aim to drink at least 1 - 2 litres throughout the day. Workout water doesn't count. Thirst is the last sign of dehydration, not the first, and indicates that you would have dehydrated at least half an hour beforehand. The body also sometimes mistakes hunger with dehydration so stave off false hunger pangs and drink up!

Rate Of Perceived Exertion (R.P.E.)

In the absence of a heart rate monitor, *rate of perceived exertion* is a great way for you to gage your training zones for maximum workout benefits.

Aerobic means with oxygen.

Anaerobic means without oxygen.

The two things that the body needs to burn fat are *oxygen* which we breathe in through air, and *fat* which we all have stores of in our bodies. Therefore if your goal is to burn fat and you are training to a point of constant breathlessness you will be doing cardio training and burning calories but *not* fat. You will also burn yourself out!

Let's use a scale of 1 - 10:

1 = completely sedentary, i.e. sitting watching tv.

7 = pulse is raised but not to the point of breathlessness - you should be able to hold a conversation, i.e. after walking up stairs.

10 = about to collapse!

During a typical *fat burning aerobic* workout:

Warm Up: 5 - 10 minutes *R.P.E. 3 - 5* (gradually raise the pulse.)

Fat Burn: 30 - 45 minutes *R.P.E 6 - 7*

Cool Down: 5 - 10 minutes *R.P.E. 7 - 3* (gradually lower the pulse.)

During an *interval* session you work both *aerobically* and *anaerobically* (dipping in and out of your cardio *and* fat burning zones)

It's all about the H.I.I.T (*High Intensity Interval Training*) circuits!

Tip: As your fitness levels increase you can decrease the warm up and increase the 'hi – lo' bursts.

Warm Up: 15 - 20 minutes *R.P.E. 3 - 7* (gradually raise the pulse.)

Raise: 1 - 2 minutes *R.P.E. 8-9 maximum* (gradually increase duration and intensity.)

Recover: 1 - 3 minutes *R.P.E. 6- 7*

Repeat the 'raise and recover' pattern for 10 - 20 minutes.

Cool Down: 5 - 10 minutes *R.P.E. 9/8/7-3* (gradually lower the pulse.)

<u>Back To Basics</u>

Though hereditary factors play a part, the most common causes of back problems are bad posture and bad habits!

The three main conditions are:

'Lordosis' which is when the pelvis tilts forward due to an exaggerated positioning in the lower back. This is frequently seen in pregnant women whose centre of balance changes due to the increased weight in the abdomen. Overweight people suffer from similar lower back ache in the sciatic region for the same reason and sciatica can also develop causing pain in the hip and calf as the sciatic nerve is connected to the hip, runs down the back of the leg and connects to the fourth toe.

'Scoliosis' which is an 'S' or 'C' shaped curvature of the spine. This is usually genetic and can be corrected with a back brace or surgery. I have scoliosis and have had none of the above and maintain a healthy spine and excellent posture through Pilates, aerobic, strength and stretch sessions, a daily supplement called Glucosamine Sulphate which is excellent for the joints, and I always have Arnica balm handy which is a natural muscle relaxant.

'Kyphosis' which causes a rounded shoulder appearance. This is common in sedentary elderly people and people who spend large periods of time in a 'hunched' position, for example at a desk. When this occurs there is usually a tightening across the chest as the muscle shortens due to poor posture, and there is additional strain on the trapezius (muscle which runs across the back of the neck and in between the shoulder blades.)

Tip: Sleep flat without a pillow so that the spine can realign and lengthen whilst releasing pressure on the neck. Pregnant women or people suffering with lower back pain like sciatica can sleep on their side with a pillow propped between the knees to keep the hips parallel and pressure off the lower spine.

All of these conditions can be treated with regular exercise and posture awareness (for example not carrying a heavy bag on your shoulder, not standing with one hip jutted out to the side, not slouching, etc.)

Tip: To find your 'neutral' or natural spine position, always stand with your 3 main planes stacked, head over ribcage and ribcage over pelvis. Never sit if you can stand, and never lie if you can sit! Also be aware of your feet as they can be pronated or supinated, which means that weight is taken on either the inside or the outside of the foot which disrupts the posture and puts pressure on the ankles, knees and spine as these areas are then forced to overcompensate to redress the balance. Look at the soles of your shoes and you will be able to see if they are worn down more on the inside or the outside. Orthotics can also help but need to be worn all the time. When standing, imagine a triangle on the soles of the feet with the points running from the heel up to the big toe and across to the little toe and try to keep your weight evenly balanced across these 3 points to bring the body back into balance. Think of the feet as tripods.

Other than pregnancy weight, it is advisable to never carry excess weight in your abdomen as this places unnecessary strain on your back. It is important to develop overall core strength.

The *general* 'core' is the rectus abdominus, obliques, transversus abdominus (the corset of muscle which runs around the waist,) the erector spinae, spine extensors, glutes, hip flexors and hip extensors. To achieve body balance it is important to mobilise, strenghten and stretch *all* of your muscles. Muscles work in pairs, yet this fact is often neglected with people overtraining the area they wish to improve, for example doing hundreds of crunches to sculpt the abs but no spinal work.

Pilates breathing for men and women: Inhale into the belly which will expand on account of the diaphragm opening Imagine a balloon in your ribcage inflating as you breathe in and deflating as you breathe out. As you exhale 'zip and hollow' (imagine that you are lacing up a corset and doing up a tight pair of trousers pulling the ribcage in and the navel tight to the back creating a dome like shape in the core.) Also engage the pelvic muscle on exhalation by lifting up internally as if you were stopping the flow of water midstream. Never *actually* do this whilst passing water as it can cause urinary infections.

Stress accumulates in the calves. The 'fight or flight' effect of adrenaline on the body in times of stress causes the calves to tense in order to prepare the body for fight or flight (remember that the body has not evolved from caveman times.) This in turn causes the body weight to shift forward onto the toes and out of alignment. The muscles remain tense as they wait to be used causing stiffness in the back. Stretching the calves and making a conscience effort to be posture aware will eliminate avoidable back aches, as will eliminating and avoiding stress in general!

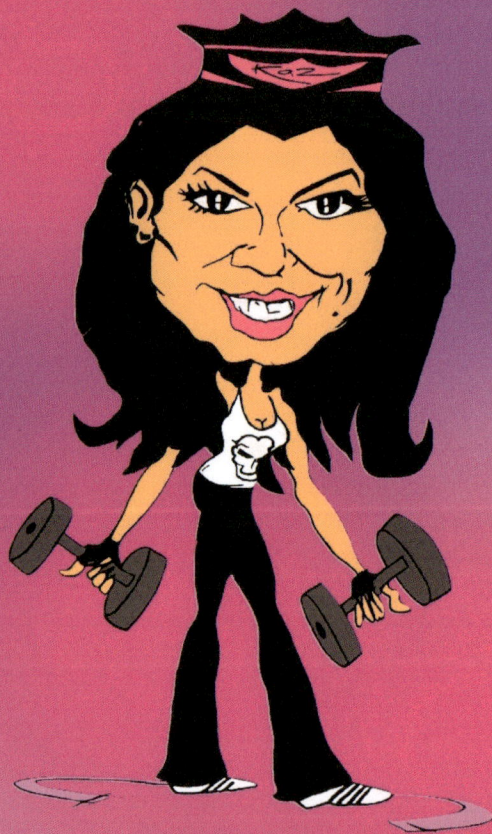

Heavy Metal

Heavy Metal!

I love dumbbells! You engage more muscle fibres, utilise core strength and raise your posture awareness through having to stabilise positions yourself in the absence of having a machine to rely on.

Women 1 - 3 kg, men 5 kg +.

Remember to exhale on the 'doing' or hardest phase, and inhale on the recovery phase, for example, on an overhead press exhale as you straighten the arms and inhale as you lower.

You should seek medical advice before beginning this or any other exercise programme, particularly if you are pregnant or have a history of medical episodes. If you are asthmatic, have your inhaler nearby - it is better to have it and not need it. Sip water before, during and after training. Increase intensity gradually, never sacrifice safety or form and always work at a level that is appropriate for *you.*

Always warm up for 5 - 10 minutes by marching/jogging on the spot, walking, doing heel digs and shallow squats, mobilise the shoulders by rolling them backwards then forwards. Close and open the arms to warm the chest. Mobilise the spine by doing twists (keep the hips facing forward and twist the torso to the right, centre, left, centre) side bends (hips and chest forward, keep the hips parallel and bend to the right side, recover, left side recover, looking in the direction you're bending in to release the neck.) Perform all movements in a controlled manner, if anything causes you discomfort stop the exercise immediately. Make sure you have your back straight and your navel pulled in to engage the core and keep your spine protected.

Tip: Warming up reduces the risk of injury, prevents Acidosis (the build up of acid in the cells which causes the muscle to prematurely fatigue) and releases muscular tension, resulting in a safer, more effective workout.

Squats (quads, hamstrings,calves,glutes, core)

Stand with the feet hip width apart. Inhale as you bend the knees - 'sit down,' thighs parallel with the floor, exhale as you stand up without locking out the knees. Hold dumbbells by your sides - the extra weight overloads the exercise and makes the muscles work harder. (15 - 20. Do 2 - 3 sets.)

Option

Deadlift (back,quads, hamstrings, calves, glutes, core))

Place dumbbells on the floor in front of you. Inhale as you bend the knees, pick up the dumbbells, exhale stand up, keeping the arms straight, hold onto the weights, each time you squat let the weights touch the floor but don't place them down until you have finished the set. (15 - 20. Do 2 - 3 sets.)

Upright Row (upper back, rear shoulders, biceps)

Stand with the feet hip width apart, knees slightly soft holding weights in front of your thighs. Exhale and lift the weights straight up the midline of the body in a vertical line aiming the elbows towards the ears and the weights towards the chin. Inhale as you straighten the arms without locking out the elbows (10 - 15. Do 2 -3 sets.)

Option

Bent Over Single Row (upper back, rear shoulder, biceps)

Rest 1 knee and hand on a bench, or you can stand with 1 leg forward, hand resting on thigh and fold forward so that your chest is parallel with the floor. With other arm, exhale and pull up - imagine that you are starting a lawnmower - aiming the elbow towards the ceiling and inhale as you straighten the arm without locking out the elbow. (10 – 15 then change arms. Do 2 -3 sets.)

Static Lunges (quads, hamstrings,hips, calves, core)

Imagine that you are standing on train tracks with a gap between your legs, back straight – think of a string attached to the top of your head lifting you up - and abdominals engaged. Take the right leg behind you and come up onto the ball of the right foot. Make sure your left knee is directly over your ankle. Inhale as you lower the right knee down to the floor in a vertical line and inhale as you recover to the starting position. If you feel discomfort in your knees, reduce your range of movement. Focus on working the rear hip flexor as this will ensure that your body is 'stacked' in correct alignment. (10 - 15 then change legs. Do 2 - 3 sets.)

Option

Alternate Lunges Forward (quads, hamstrings,hips, calves, core, cardiovascular)

Start with feet together. Step forward on the right leg, heel lands first, knee over ankle and back straight. Inhale as you lower knee to the ground, exhale as you recover and return to the starting position. Change sides. (10 - 15. Do 2 - 3 sets.)

Option

Alternate Lunges Backwards (quads, hamstring, hips, calves, core, cardiovascular)

Start with feet together. Step backwards on the right leg landing on the ball of the foot; keeping the left knee over the ankle and the back straight. Inhale as you lower knee to the ground, exhale as you recover and return to the starting position. Change sides. (10 - 15 on each leg. Do 2 - 3 sets.)

Bicep Curls (fronts of arms)

This exercise can be performed either sitting or standing. Start with the arms at the side of the body, turned slightly out on the diagonal. This will recruit the middle (belly) of the muscle as there are 3 heads. Keep the upper arms close to the ribcage. Exhale as you bend the arms bringing the weights towards the shoulders. Imagine that you are crushing a walnut in the crease of the forearm. Exhale as you straighten the arms without locking out the elbows. (10 - 15. Do 2 - 3 sets.)

Option

Single Seated Bicep Curl (front of arm)

Let the nonworking hand rest on thigh. Rest elbow on the thigh, arm coming between your legs lean your body slightly forward. Exhale as you curl, inhale as you straighten the arm. In this position, you won't straighten the arm completely on return. (10 – 15 then change arms. Do 2 - 3 sets.)

Overhead Press (shoulders, upper back, triceps, core)

This exercise can also be performed either sitting or standing. Hold the weights horizontally at shoulder level, palms facing forward. Exhale as you straighten the arms above the head without locking out the elbows, and try not to arch the back. Inhale as you recover. (10 - 15. Do 2 - 3 sets.)

Option

Alternate Single Shoulder Press (shoulders, upper back, triceps, core)

As above, but do 1 arm at a time and alternate after each repetition. (10 - 15. Do 2 - 3 sets.)

Chest Press (chest, shoulders, triceps, core)

Lie down, abdominals tight and back tight to the bench/floor. If you are on the floor, have your knees bent and your feet placed hip width apart. Hold the weights horizontally at chest level, knuckles towards the ceiling. Exhale as you straighten the arms without locking out the elbow. Inhale as you recover. (15 - 20. Do 2 - 3 sets.)

Tricep Extensions (backs of arms)

Once again you can sit or stand for this exercise. Bend the arms so that the dumbbells are behind the head and the elbows are going vertically towards the ceiling. Keeping the elbows stationary, exhale as you straighten the arms towards the ceiling without arching the back or locking out the elbows. Inhale as you recover. (10 - 15. Do 2 - 3 sets.)

Option

Single Tricep Extensions (back of arm)

As above but do 1 arm at a time. Working arm can be held and stabilised if required (10 - 15. Do 2 - 3 sets.)

Side Leg Lifts (hips, outer thigh)

Lie down on your side with your hips parallel and the legs in line with the upper body. Head can rest on the arm or in the hand. Exhale as you lift the upper leg towards the ceiling keeping the inner thigh down to the floor - no outward rotation in the hip. Inhale as you return to the starting position. (15 - 20. Do 2 - 3 sets.)

Inner Thighs

Lie down on your back and straighten your legs towards the ceiling so that your feet are directly over the hips. Inhale as you open the legs, exhale and imagine that you are squeezing against a resistance as you close. Keep your knees straight and if you need to break at any point draw your knees into your chest. If you need additional support for your lower back place your hands under your hips.

(15 - 20. Do 2 - 3 sets.)

Tip: Bigger muscles and muscle groups need more weight/repetitions.

Increase your weights when the exercise starts becoming too easy and reduce the sets and build up gradually again. Don't waste your workout doing 'junk repetitions' – make each one count on their own merit. If you are sitting down for upper body work, try using a stability ball to further challenge the core. To keep things fresh and avoid plateau, mix things up by doing exercises in a different sequence, for example upper body then lower body, then upper body etc which will also keep the heart rate up. Another option would be to warm up and then do this programme in reverse order. Remember to realign your muscle fibres by stretching afterwards for 10 - 45 seconds on each muscle worked.

Tip: The bicep stretch (face palm away then gently pull fingers towards the elbow) helps to avoid RSI (Repetitive Strain Injury) so do it periodically if doing long spells of typing, driving, playing a musical instrument, etc.

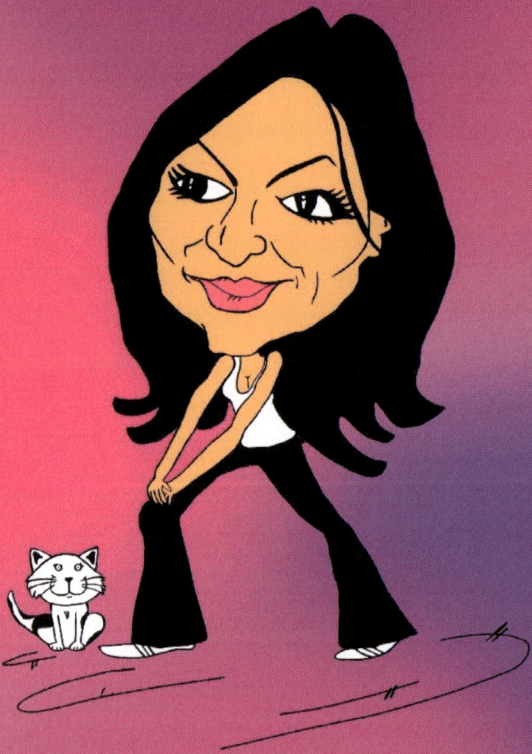

Calf Stretch

I Am Too Busy To Cook Healthy Dinners!

No more excuses with these 20 minute or less from 'stove to stomach' mouth-watering concoctions!

Chinese Stir Fry

Spray a pan with low calorie oil spray or fry in water. Add fresh or frozen onion, peppers, cauliflower, green beans, sweet corn and carrots. Season with garlic, a dash of soy sauce and chilli flakes. Stir fry for 10 - 15 minutes or until the vegetables are soft.

Serve with grilled fish, prawns or tofu.

Marinade for fish, prawns or tofu

Garlic, ginger, lemon/lime slice, balsamic vinegar, ground black pepper, agave nectar or honey. Grill or dry fry for 10 - 15 minutes turning occasionally.

Kaz's Kick Ass Kurry (choose from either quorn -fresh or frozen- prawns, chick peas or soya beans) MEAT FREE AND WHEAT FREE

Spray a pan with low calorie oil spray or fry in water. Add fresh or frozen onion, spinach, peppers and canned tomatoes. Season with garlic, ginger, coriander, cumin, cayenne pepper, 1 tsp of tomato ketchup, 1 tblsp of curry powder and 1 tsp of madras curry paste (adjust the amounts depending on how hot /mild you like your curry.) Stir fry until the vegetables are soft. Add chosen filling and simmer for a further 10 minutes or until the sauce thickens.

Serve with quinoa and a dollop of natural organic yoghurt and mango chutney (optional.)

Tip: Curry tastes better when it has time to marinade!

Chilli Quorn Carne – MEAT FREE AND WHEAT FREE

Spray a pan with low calorie oil spray or fry in water. Add fresh or frozen onion and canned tomatoes. Season with garlic, cumin, chilli flakes and 1 tsp of tomato ketchup. Stir fry until onions are soft. Add quorn (fresh or frozen) and a can of kidney beans (rinsed and drained.) Simmer for a further 10 minutes or until the sauce thickens.

Serve with quinoa.

Egg White Omelettes

Spray a non stick pan with low calorie oil spray.

Remove yolk from 1 egg – use 2, and then whisk in a bowl until frothy or you can buy egg whites already prepared. Fry onions, mushrooms, peppers or vegetables first, remove from pan and then add back once the egg whites are in the pan. Add cheese if desired. Allow to cook on low heat, fold in half, and turn over once.

Serve with salad and baked beans.

Black Bean Burrito and Guacamole Dip

Scramble 2 egg whites with ¼ cup of black beans (rinsed and drained) 2 tblsp of salsa and 2 tblsp of cheese. Add the ingredients to 1 wholemeal tortilla.

Guacamole Dip

Add 1 chopped avocado to finely chopped tomato, ½ red onion, lime juice and chilli flakes.

Spinach & Strawberry Salad

Combine on a plate 2 cups of baby spinach, 1 cup of shredded lettuce, ½ cup of sliced strawberries, ½ cup of broccoli florets, 1 chopped hard boiled egg minus the yolk and ¼ cup of kidney beans. Drizzle with vinaigrette.

Have a well stocked spice rack so that you can create delicious meals in an instant. Invest in balsamic vinegar, white wine vinegar, olive oil, honey and agave nectar so that you can make marinades and salad dressings. Keep your freezer stocked with frozen vegetables and fish fillets, prawns and quorn. Quorn is high in protein, low in fat and a fantastic, ethical alternative to meat. You can freeze wholemeal pitta bread. Substitute normal potatoes with sweet potatoes which have a lower G.I. level and are high in vitamin C. They are delicious baked or made into chunky chips! Have sunflower and pumpkin seeds for snacks and sprinkle them on salads and soups (use sparingly as they can be calorific.) Use skimmed organic milk or almond, soya or rice milk instead of whole milk. Replace beer and wine which are carbohydrates with spirits and low fat mixers.

Cook large batches of food so that some can be frozen for a later date.

*A*pples - 2 daily lower cholesterol levels by 10 per cent. They are a great source of fibre, iron and vitamin C and are beneficial for the joints. Good for arthritis, rheumatism and gout.

*B*lueberries - powerful antioxidant and high in vitamin C.

Cranberries - vitamin A and C. High in iron and potassium. Good for flushing out urinary tract infections.

Dates - high in fibre and potassium.

E – vitamin, found in avocado along with vitamins A, B and C. One avocado a week balances hormones in women, sheds birth weight and can prevent cervical cancer. Good for glowing skin and hair and has anti ageing benefits.

Fusion - of mind, body and spirit for overall well being!

Green Tea - antioxidant and boosts metabolism. It contains an amino acid called L-thiamine which increases alpha brain waves resulting in relaxation of the body and mind.

Hazelnuts - high in magnesium, phosphorus and thiamine.

Jalapeno - cayenne and chilli peppers boost metabolism. Good for the respiratory system as excess debris is shifted from the lungs.

Kidney beans - help to heal and maintain kidney function.

Lycopene - found in tomatoes along with vitamins C and E. Tomatoes are excellent heart and blood food and prevent some forms of cancer, particularly prostate.

*M*ushrooms - high in protein and B12.

*N*uts - and seeds, great form of omega fat.

*O*nions - remove toxins from the body.

*P*runes - high in potassium which lowers high blood pressure and rich in fibre, iron, vitamins A and B6.

*Q*uinoa –great alternative for starchy carbohydrates like rice and pasta and a good source of protein.

*R*hubarb - targets bone strength and replenishes the skeletal needs.

*S*trawberries - eliminate kidney stones, lower blood pressure and are high in iron. Good for arthritis, rheumatism and gout.

*T*wenty minutes - the time it takes for your brain to register that your stomach is full so slow down!

*U*FO - unidentified food object! Try to avoid foods laden with additives and preservatives. Read the label.

*V*ital - essential fatty acids. Your body needs them but cannot make them so they must be obtained from food. Omega 3, 6, and 9 are compulsory for cardiovascular health, and are found in fatty fish, olive oil, hemp seed oil, nuts, seeds and avocados. They can also be taken in a supplement form. A 'chicken skin' appearance on the upper arms (keratosis pilaris, 'KP') could be an indication of a lack of essential fatty acid when keratin (a protein found in skin hair and nails) builds up in the skin follicles causing rough raised bumps to appear on the surface. This occurs when there is a lack of sebum (natural lubrication oil for the skin) which disrupts the natural skin shedding process resulting in clogged pores.

*W*alnuts – contain acids which convert into Omega 3 fat. Also high in protein, potassium, zinc and iron.

*X*tra - unwanted portions and calories!

*Y*es - to positive life enhancing changes!

*Z*inc - found in pumpkin and sesame seeds, shellfish (especially oysters) wheat germ, cheese, and eggs. Assists with production of collagen which gives skin its elasticity.

No Time? No Problem! No Nonsense Power Breakfasts

Peanut Butter and Banana Smoothie

¼ pint of organic skimmed, soya, almond or rice milk, 1 tsp of organic peanut butter, 1 medium banana, ice cubes and a scoop of protein powder. Combine using either a blender or hand whisk.

Blueberry & Toasted Almond & Walnut Muesli

Pour ½ cup organic skimmed, soya, almond or rice milk over ½ cup of oats and allow to sit for 10 minutes or combine the milk and oats and keep it in the fridge overnight. Add ½ cup of blueberries, 1 tbsp of almonds and 1 tblsp of walnuts.

Granola (8 servings)

Mix in a large bowl 4 cups of rolled oats, ½ cup of raisins, ½ cup of goji berries, 6 chopped apricots and 4 tblsp of honey or agave nectar and then place in a non stick baking tray.

Bake for 25 minutes, and then remove the mixture and stir. Bake for a further 15 minutes or until the granola is crisp and golden brown. Delicious hot or cold, on its own or with organic skimmed, soya, almond or rice milk or natural yoghurt.

Quinoa Porridge

In a pan bring 1 cup of quinoa, 2 cups of almond milk and ½ tsp of vanilla to the boil. Simmer until the liquid is absorbed (15 – 20 minutes.). Garnish with a sprinkling of cinnamon or/and fruit if desired.

Slimline Breakfast Pizza

Spread tomato puree onto Ryvita or other cracker bread.
Add grated cheese, sliced mushrooms and sliced
tomatoes. Grill until cheese bubbles.

BBP (Big Breakfast Pitta)

Toast 1 wholemeal pitta bread. Cut into 2 halves.
Separate and stuff with 1 scrambled egg, grilled or dry
fried mushroom and tomato and garnish with cheese and
tomato ketchup.

Shopping List

Cupboard

Rolled oats

Raisins

Goji berries

Apricots

Almonds

Walnuts

Dates

Sunflower seeds

Pumpkin seeds

Balsimic vinegar

Organic apple cider vinegar

Light soy sauce

Olive oil

Low calorie cooking oil spray

Quinoa

Brown rice

Chilli flakes

Cayenne pepper

Madras Curry Paste

Ryvita

Tomato ketchup

Tomato puree

Honey

Agave nectar

Ground black pepper

Tinned tomatoes

Tinned sweetcorn

Tinned tuna

Tinned mackerel

Tinned sardines

Tinned baked beans

Tinned black beans

Tinned kidney beans

Tinned fruit (in natural juice)

Organic peanut butter

Fresh

Organic skimmed, soya, almond or rice milk

Natural organic yoghurt

Organic eggs

Fish

Prawns

Quorn

Organic cottage cheese

Feta cheese

Mozzarella

Mixed salad leaves (pre prepared)

Spinach (washed and ready to eat)

Garlic

Ginger

Lemons

Limes

Bananas

Apples

Seasonal fruit

Seasonal vegetables

Wholemeal pitta (can be frozen)

Wholemeal tortilla (can be frozen)

Sweet potatoes

Mineral water

Cranberry juice

Pomegranate juice

Orange juice

Tip: Don't buy fruit juice made from concentrate. Try juicing carrots and then add *fresh* orange juice to save time.

Frozen

Mixed berries (great for smoothies or desserts when served with natural yoghurt, honey and sprinkled with sunflower seeds.

Vegetables (peas, carrots, sweet corn, green beans etc.)

Tip: Vegetables are frozen within hours of being harvested and therefore maintain their vital nutrients. You use the exact amount required as needed and so avoid waste. Wash fresh fruit and vegetables where applicable to remove pesticides and soil (particularly important for pregnant women as they are susceptible to toxoplasmosis. On that note, if relevant, pregnant women should also wear gloves and wash their hands thoroughly if handling cat litter.)

A tablespoon of organic apple cider vinegar daily reduces bloat in the abdomen and flushes toxins from the body.

Food Diary (Please complete all sections daily)

Monday

Breakfast

Lunch

Dinner

Snacks

Activity

Tuesday

Breakfast

Lunch

Dinner

Snacks

Activity

Wednesday

Breakfast

Lunch

Dinner

Snacks

Activity

Thursday

Breakfast

Lunch

Dinner

Snacks

Activity

Friday

Breakfast

Lunch

Dinner

Snacks

Activity

Saturday

Breakfast

Lunch

Dinner

Snacks

Activity

Sunday

Breakfast

Lunch

Dinner

Snacks

Activity

The 4 P Programme

Protein

Replenishes muscle fibre, blunts appetite and builds a lean, sculpted physique.

Drink plenty of water and don't overdo it – you're looking at 1 lb of protein for each lb of body weight. The body can only absorb approximately 20 - 30grams at once though this varies slightly depending on body type, activity, training needs etc.

Sources include organic egg whites, cottage cheese, yoghurt, skimmed milk, pulses and protein shakes.

Plyometrics

Plyometrics or 'jump training' – fantastic for revving up the metabolism as it raises the heart rate to work you at your maximum capacity. Great in circuits when you can alternate between high and low intensity levels and recover in between bursts.

Planks

Moving or static – all are whole body and engage the core to rip the abs.

Pilates

Pilates elongates and strengthens the whole body and focuses on core muscle groups. It compliments the more high impact classes by allowing the body to recover whilst still working and works wonders for people with back problems.

I Can Get the Life I Want When I Am Thin

Tip: Do 1 thing every day that makes you happy. Write it down. That is all.

You can start getting the life you want right now! Whilst an upcoming event can be a great motivation to address any body issues you may have, you cannot and should not exile yourself until you are 'thin.' It is true that inch and weight loss does wonders for your self esteem as looking good equals feeling good, especially when you have worked hard at achieving it. Success breeds success. That mindset can be applied to any life goal. Bad habits are *learned*, and therefore can be *reversed* and *replaced* with a more positive attitude. All the while you think that you don't deserve the 'perfect' job, relationship, house, or social life until you look a certain way you are reaffirming the old negative beliefs that kept you locked in the binge/starvation zone in the first place. Many of us have used food to medicate our feelings at some point which has been the problem - the *relationship* we've had with the food, not the *food* itself. Excess weight is the symptom, not the cause. We are looking at positive life changes, not a 6 week whim. We know that diets don't work. The only 'perfect' food and exercise plan for you is 1 that *you* can stick to. There is no magic answer, but then we are not dealing with rocket science here. Wisdom is, after all, seeing the same old situation in a brand new way. In the majority of cases, it's not that people don't know what to do. They just don't do it!

Tip: 'If you're doing something wrong, doing it more intensely isn't going to help.' *Vince Lombardi - American Football Coach.*

I have worked as a fittings model and can tell you first hand that things are rarely as they seem. For example, clothes are cut 1cm bigger and 1cm smaller on garments of the same size so you get the same 'size' in bigger and smaller versions. The images we see in magazines and on billboards, although amazing, have often been waved with the magic airbrushing wand, not to mention a team of excellent professionals who use styling and lighting to create the most 'perfect' models possible beforehand as well! If someone or something inspires you to run that extra mile then great, but don't be deceived. Accept your natural body shape and make it the best it can be. Above all else, be happy in your own skin! This is truly the key to success for everything in life.

Tip: When life hands you lemons, slice neatly and add to gin and (slim line) tonic. Enjoy responsibly with friends.

The End

ACKNOWLEDGEMENTS

Special thanks to my graphic designer Shuk.M for bringing everything so painstakingly to life and Geoff Lyons for the initial sketches.

XOXOXO

EXTERNAL LINKS

https://rockyourworkout.wordpress.com/

https://www.facebook.com/cantfrymelove

https://twitter.com/KARENLANSON

18861962R00047

Printed in Poland
by Amazon Fulfillment
Poland Sp. z o.o., Wrocław